Nurse Teddy Bear Learns About Food Allergies

Written by: Ann Lempert Deutsch

Illustrated by: Students with Food Allergies

DEDICATION

This book is dedicated to Dennis, Dara and Matthew, to children with food allergies, and to people everywhere who need to learn about food allergies.

School Food Allergy Guidelines

Schools recognize the growing number of students with potentially life threatening food allergies. They are committed to the safety of all of their students. As a school nurse, I recognize the responsibility to develop appropriate food allergy plans that detail emergency management and address conditions to prevent exposure to specific allergens. It is my belief that a collaborative partnership between school and family is the best way to achieve this goal while thoughtfully increasing the student's independence.

A collaborative relationship within the entire school community can provide a safe and healthy learning environment. As a result, parents and their children with food allergies will be able to make the transition between the safety of their home environment into the expanding world of school. When done well, this is one of the greatest lessons that a child with food allergies can learn. At the same time, classmates without food allergies can develop a greater understanding of individual differences along with the capacity for flexibility and increased compassion.

These suggested guidelines are intended to address the specific needs of food allergic students and the creation of a safe environment for all. Please refer to the School Food Allergy Facts, Suggested Guidelines and valuable resources at the back of this book. Although the medical and health related needs for each student are unique, the goal of these guidelines is to establish consistent practices throughout a school. It is important to note that the implementation of these guidelines will be considered in light of the developmental level of the students and may be modified to meet individual needs. Parents must always consult their physician when planning the best action to take.

Ann Lempert Deutsch

February, 2012

It was September 6th at 7 A.M. "Get up!! You'll be late for the first day of school!" said Mr. Carewell as he tried to wake Nurse Carewell up.

"A few more minutes" Nurse Carewell said. "I can't believe summer is over!

I'm not ready to start another year. It went so fast, it feels like the last day of school was only yesterday!"

"But not for me. I was so excited," said Nurse Teddy Bear. It was the first day of school and I couldn't wait to go. I had been home with Nurse Carewell all summer and now it was time to go back to school.

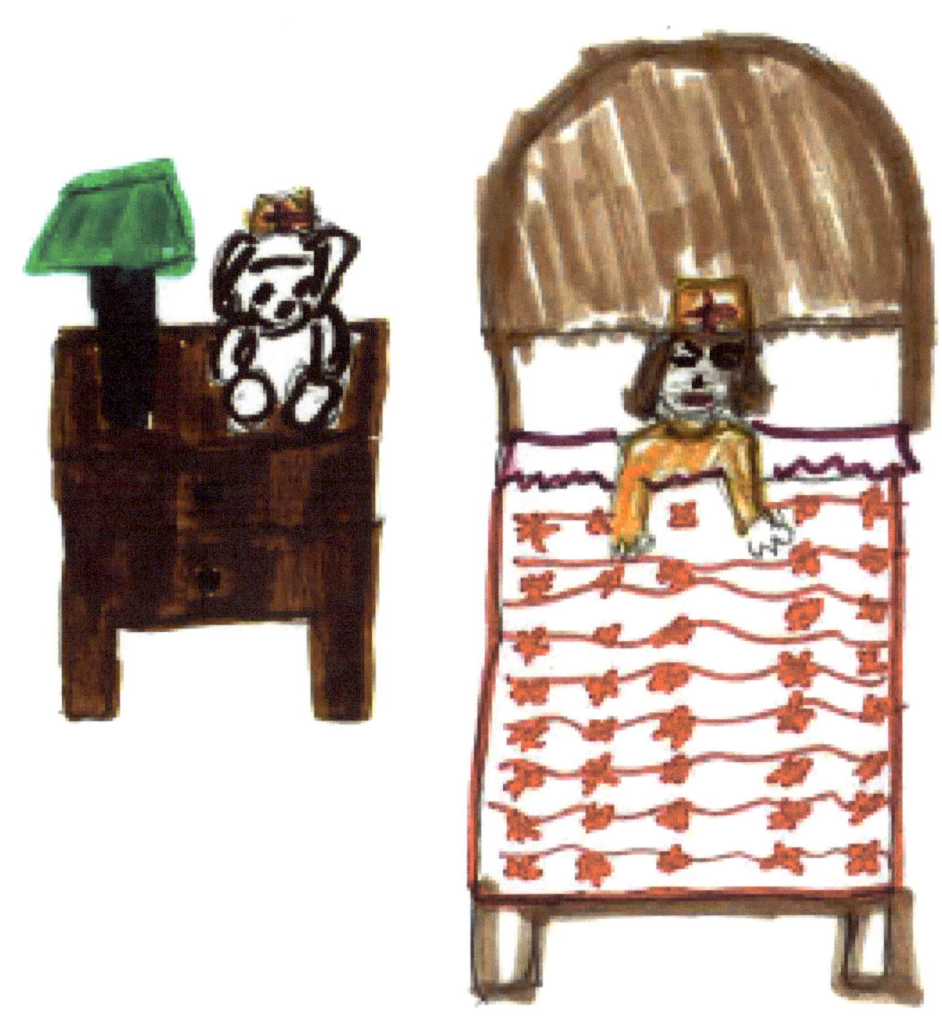

Matthew, Age 12
Allergic to all nuts except almonds

We ate breakfast, brushed our teeth and kissed everyone good-bye. We got in the car, buckled our seat belts and drove to school. Meadows Elementary School is a mile from my house.

When I arrived, I saw children outside playing, many with their new backpacks and sneakers. Nurse Carewell got out of the car. As she approached the school, she knew summer was behind her and she was ready to start another school year. She hadn't realized how much she'd missed seeing the many smiling faces of the children.

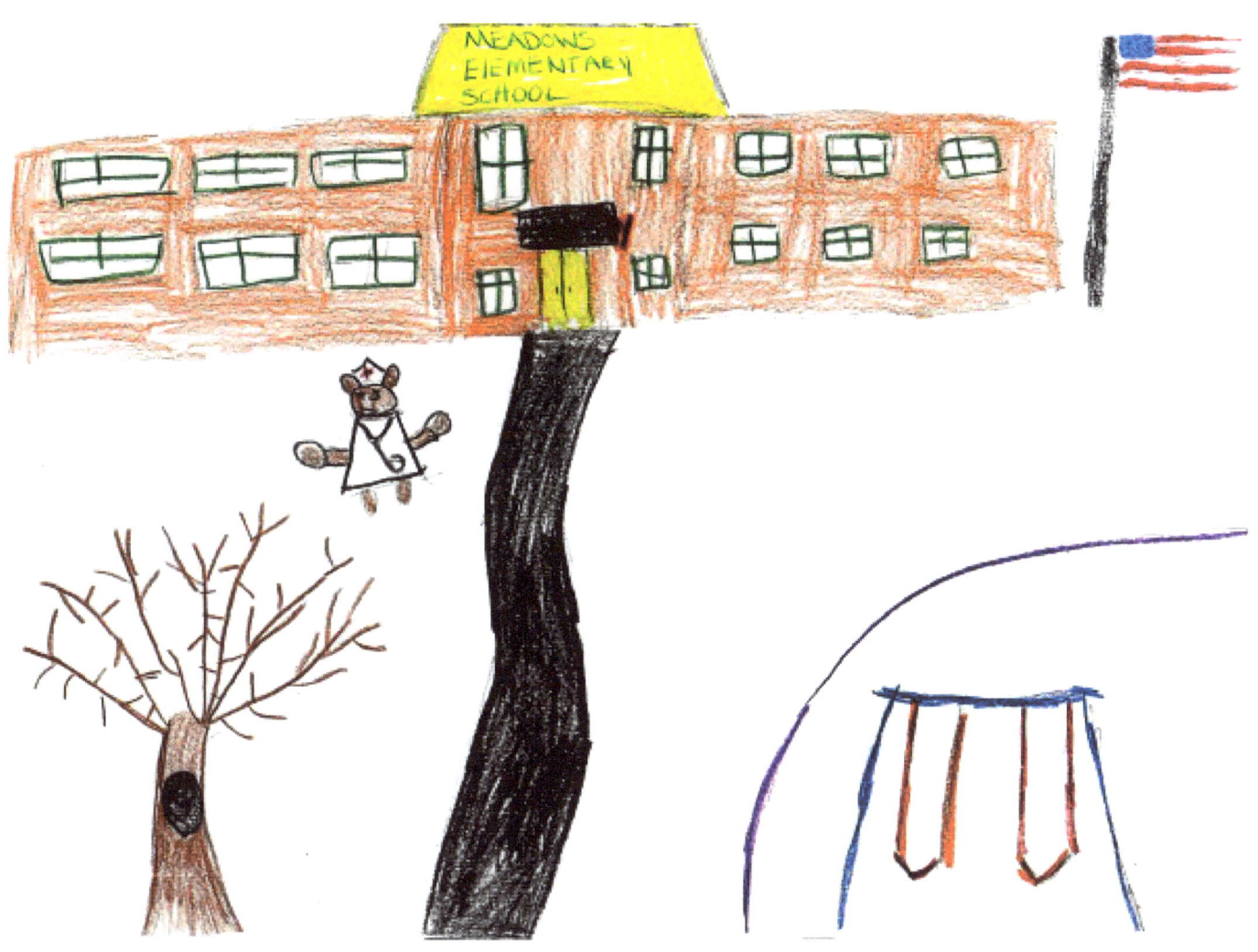

Devin, Age 10
Allergic to peanuts, tree nuts and seeds

Nurse Carewell entered the building and was greeted by a group of second graders. They looked so much older since June. "Hi, Nurse Carewell. Hi Nurse Teddy Bear."

The bell rang and a new school year began.

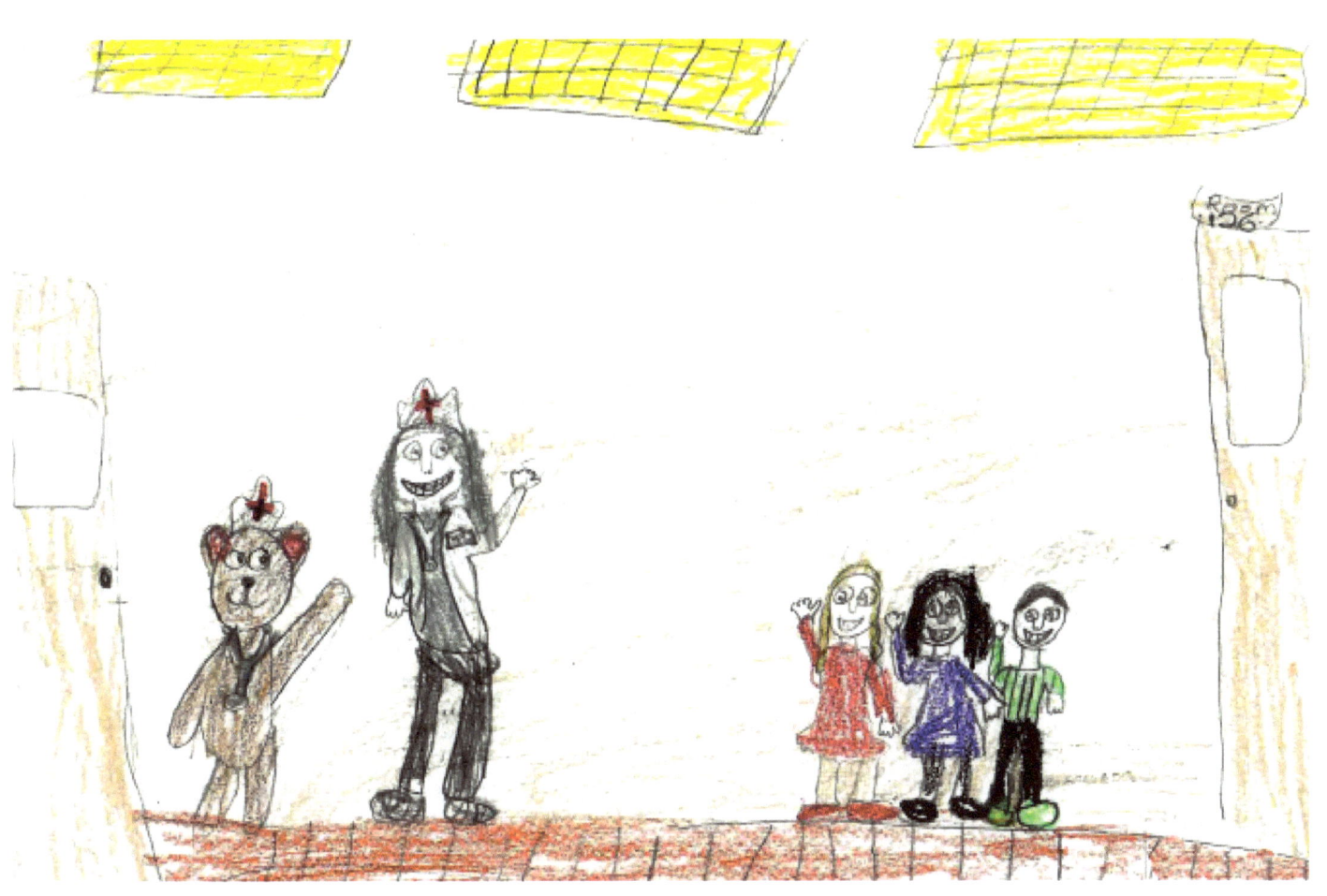

Elisabeth, Age 9
Allergic to eggs and peanuts

The morning was spent meeting new students and their parents. Many of the students walked by the Health Office and waved hello. Some stopped in briefly and told us about their summer.

Dara's mom came in to leave Dara's medicine with Nurse Carewell; Dara was allergic to peanuts and tree nuts. Nurse Carewell explained to Dara's mother that we were going to visit her class shortly to explain to the students what food allergies are.

I couldn't wait to go into the classroom and meet the students who would be taking me home.

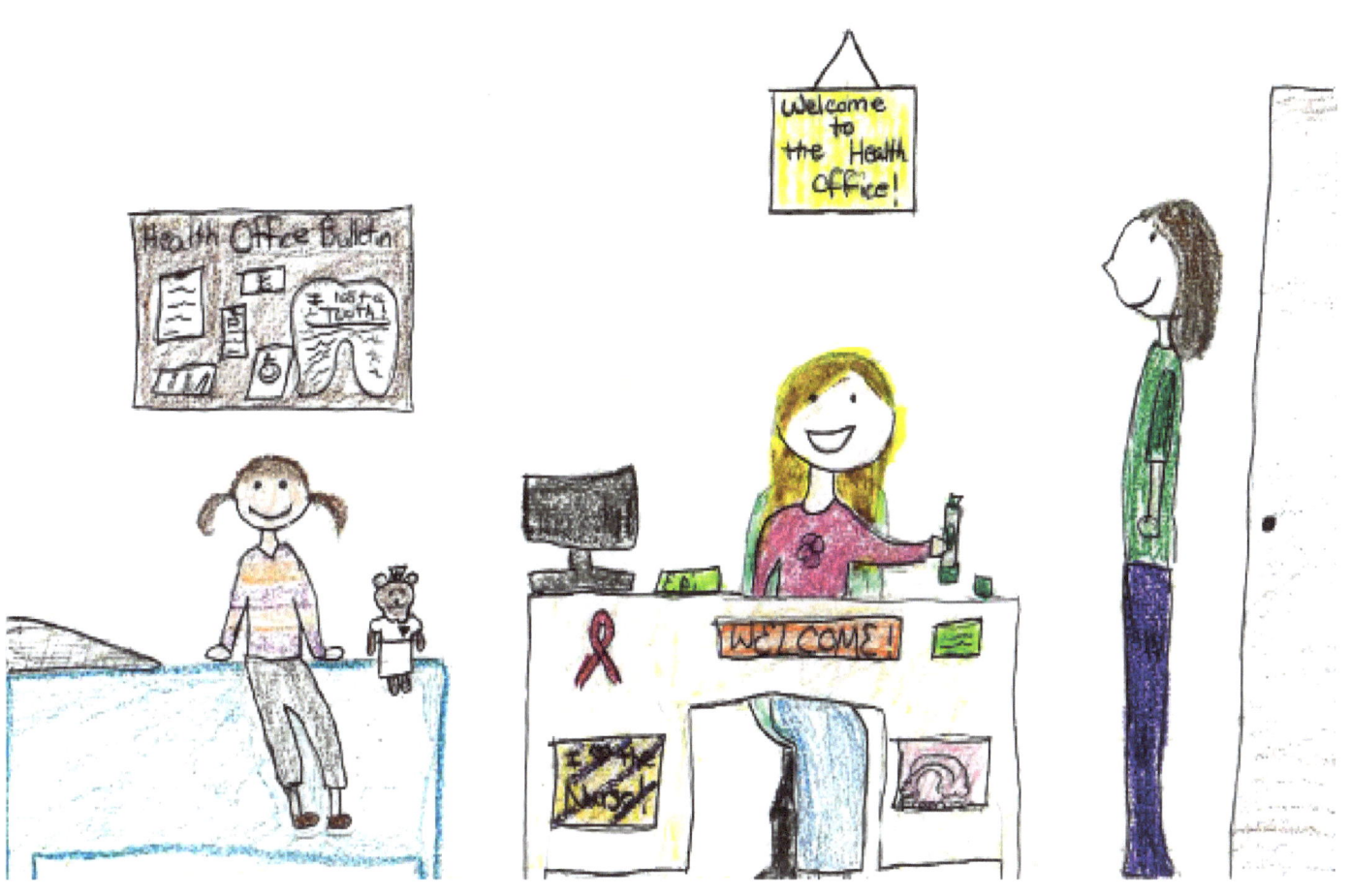

Claire, Age 10
Allergic to peanuts, tree nuts, apples and strawberries

Nurse Carewell and I went into Dara's class. Nurse Carewell explained about food allergies and compared how we fight allergies to the way our bodies fight against other harmful things such as the common cold.

She explained that sometimes our body makes a mistake and thinks a food is harmful; our body reacts by making a special substance called an "antibody" to fight that food.

The next time a child with allergies eats that food, their body releases a chemical called a "histamine" into their blood stream.

It is the body's "battle" against those histamines that causes the allergy symptoms.

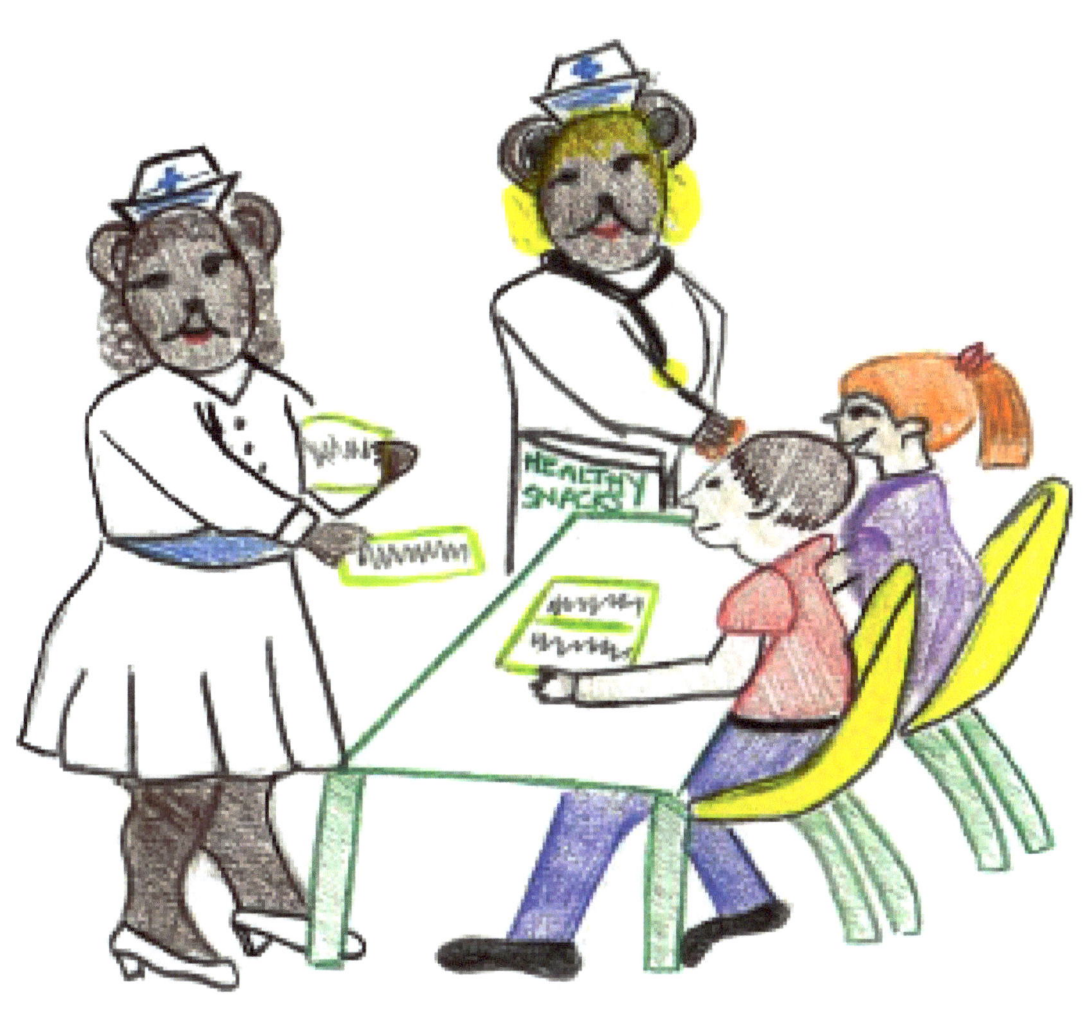

Christian, Age 12
Allergic to all nuts

There are many foods that children can be allergic to. Allergies to peanuts and tree nuts (walnuts, almonds, cashews) are common, and so are allergies to fish, eggs, milk, soy, wheat and shellfish such as shrimp.

Nurse Carewell said that when some children eat these foods it could make them sick. If they eat a food that they are allergic to, they may develop a rash, get sick to their stomach, have a funny feeling around their mouth and tongue, their lips might get swollen, and they might even have trouble breathing.

Nurse Carewell also mentioned how important it is to tell an adult right away if any of your allergy friends say they don't feel well or are acting like they're sick.

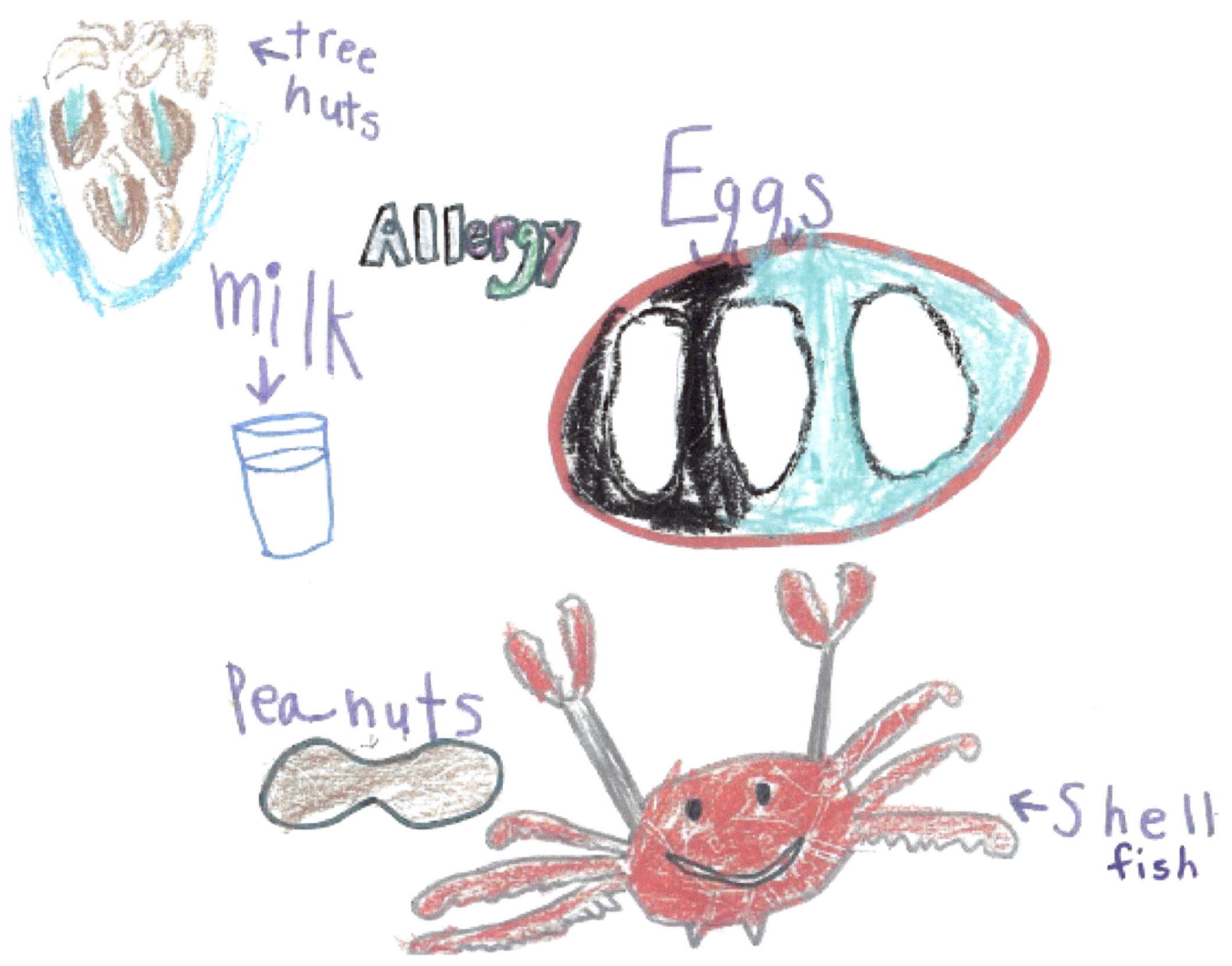

Benny, Age 6
Allergic to sesame, peanuts, tree nuts, shellfish

Then Nurse Carewell talked about sharing.

Although teachers always teach the children to be good sharers (like sharing their crayons, for example), Nurse Carewell warned them NOT to share their food.

She explained that they were in a special peanut/tree nut classroom and she did not want anyone to bring in snacks that contained peanuts or tree nuts. That way, the students who could not eat those foods would feel safe in the classroom.

I blurted out, "Food we never share."

And then Nurse Carewell said, "Listen to Nurse Teddy Bear!"

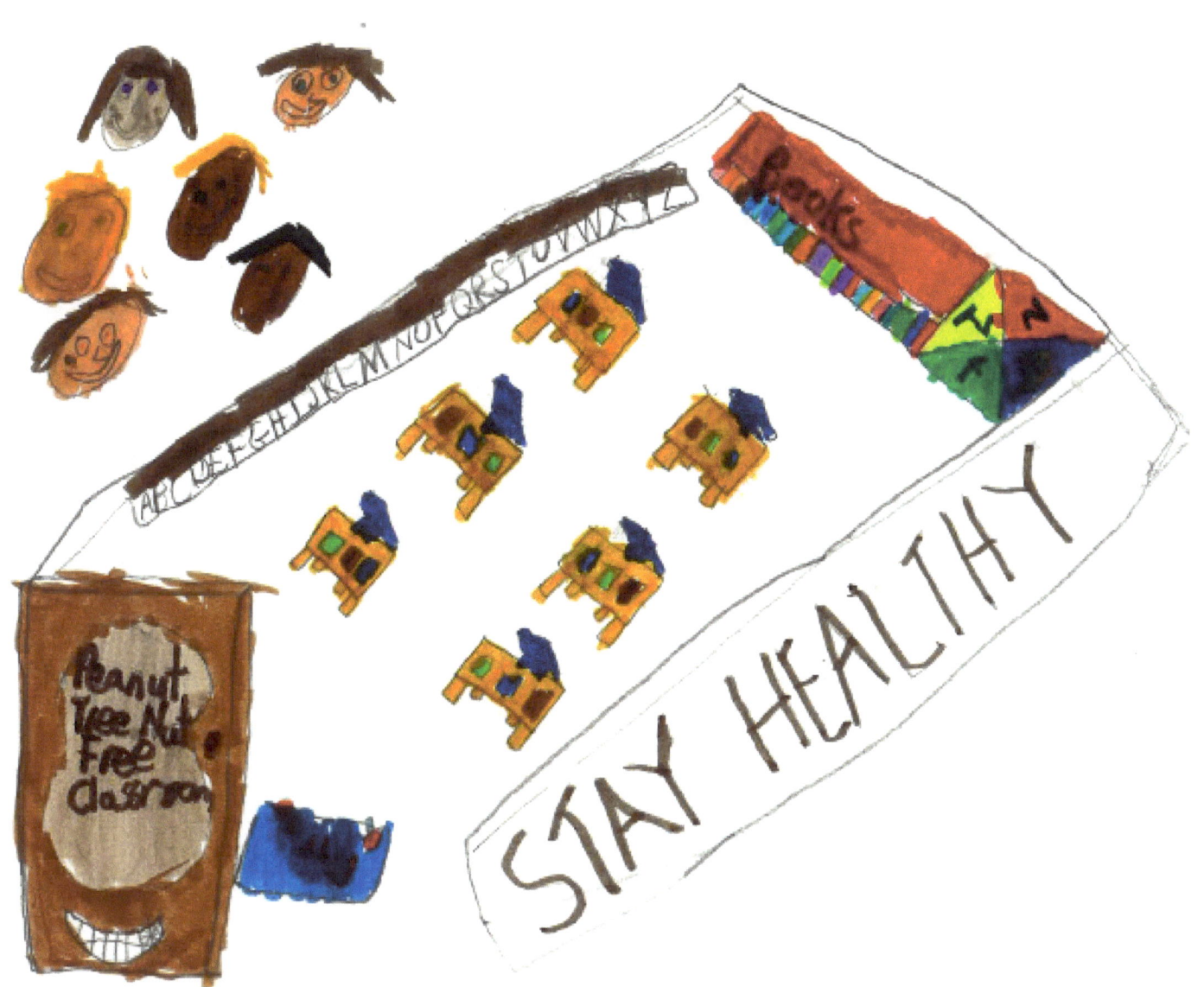

Michael, Age 9
Allergic to peanuts

Nurse Carewell also explained during lunch that there would be a special table for children with food allergies.

Each week a few students that did not have allergies could sit with their friends at the special table, but they could not bring in foods such as peanut butter and jelly sandwiches when sitting at that table.

As soon as Nurse Carewell finished explaining, the class sang out "Food we never share, listen to Nurse Teddy Bear!"

I was so excited!

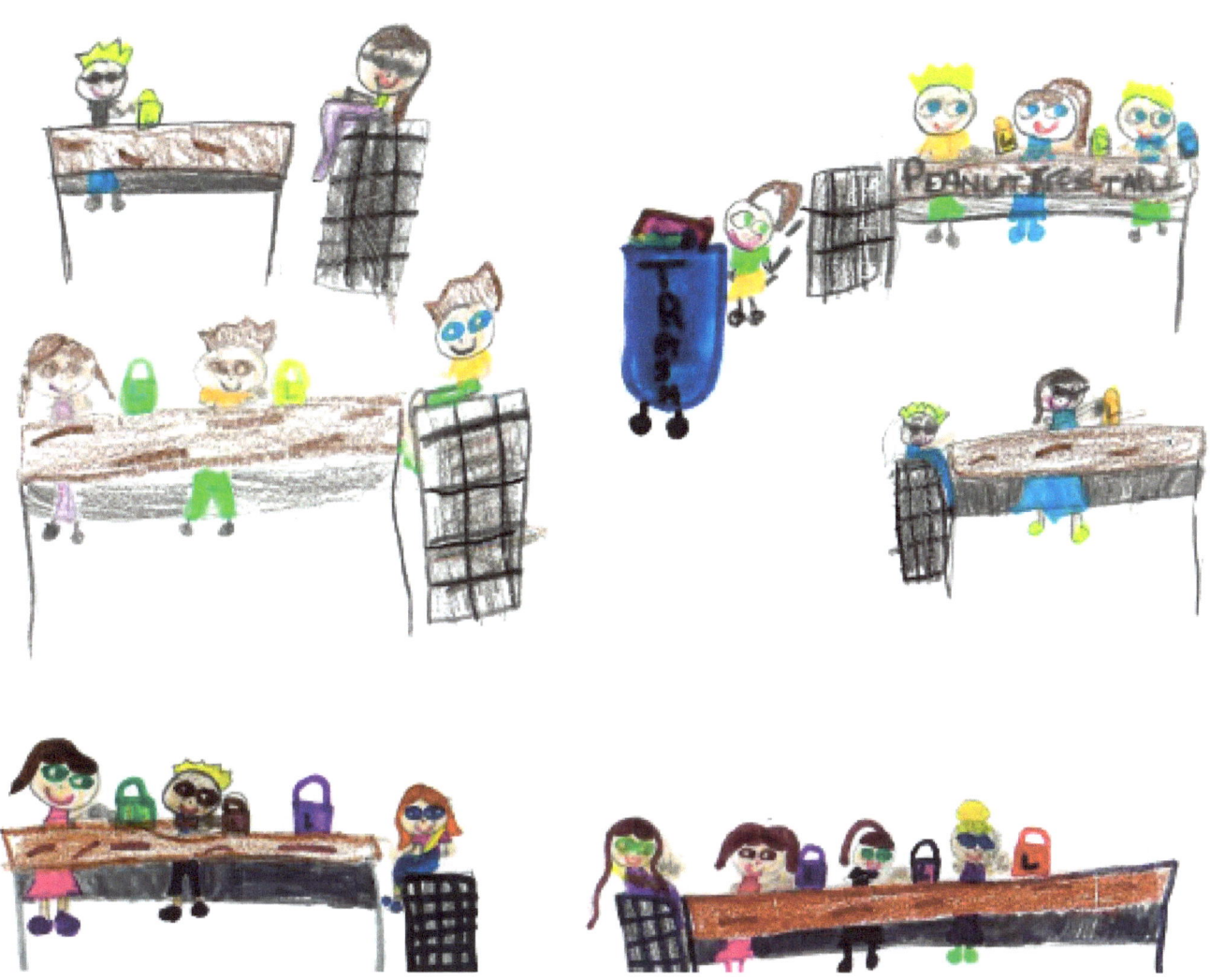

Arianna, Age 9
Allergic to mushrooms and shellfish

Then came the best part! Nurse Carewell finally introduced me to the class!

She explained that I was her helper and I was tired of just sitting around the Health Office. (This was somewhat true, but I did like watching what went on in the office!)

She explained that I would be going home with each student for a week and it was his or her job to teach me something related to health. I loved going home with students and learning healthy habits.

Nurse Carewell then said good-bye to the class and left me in the classroom. I found out later that I'd be going home with Dara this week. I couldn't wait!

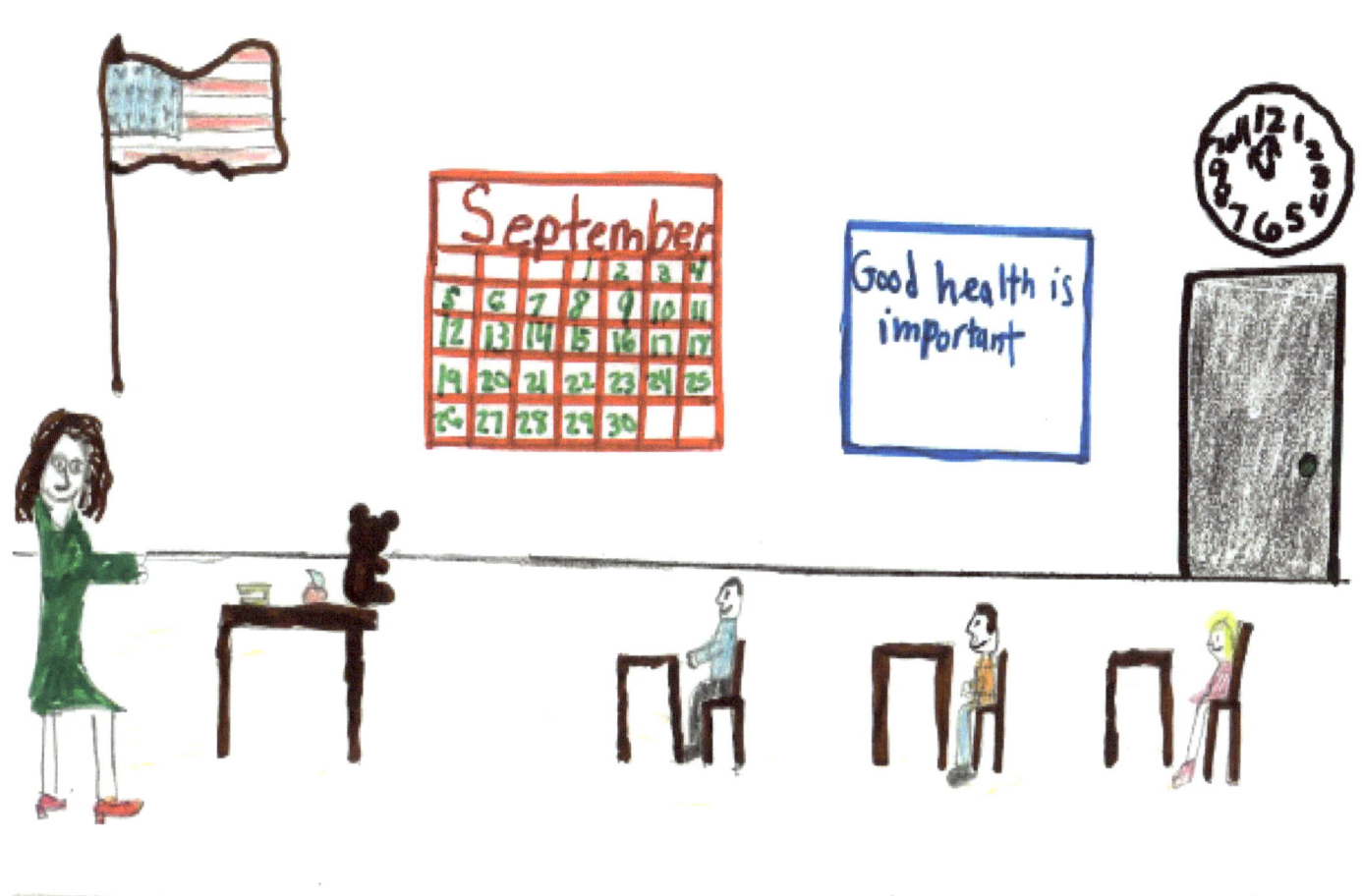

Steven, Age 9
Allergic to tree nuts

The day went by so fast that before I knew it, it was time for Dara and I to go home!

We stopped by the Health Office on our way out. Dara's mom told Nurse Carewell about Dara's first allergic reaction (to peanut butter) and how her lips had swelled up, a rash had developed around her mouth, and her tongue had started to tingle. When Dara's reaction happened, she was immediately taken to the Emergency Room where she received a shot (an injection) of epinephrine.

That shot made Dara feel better immediately!

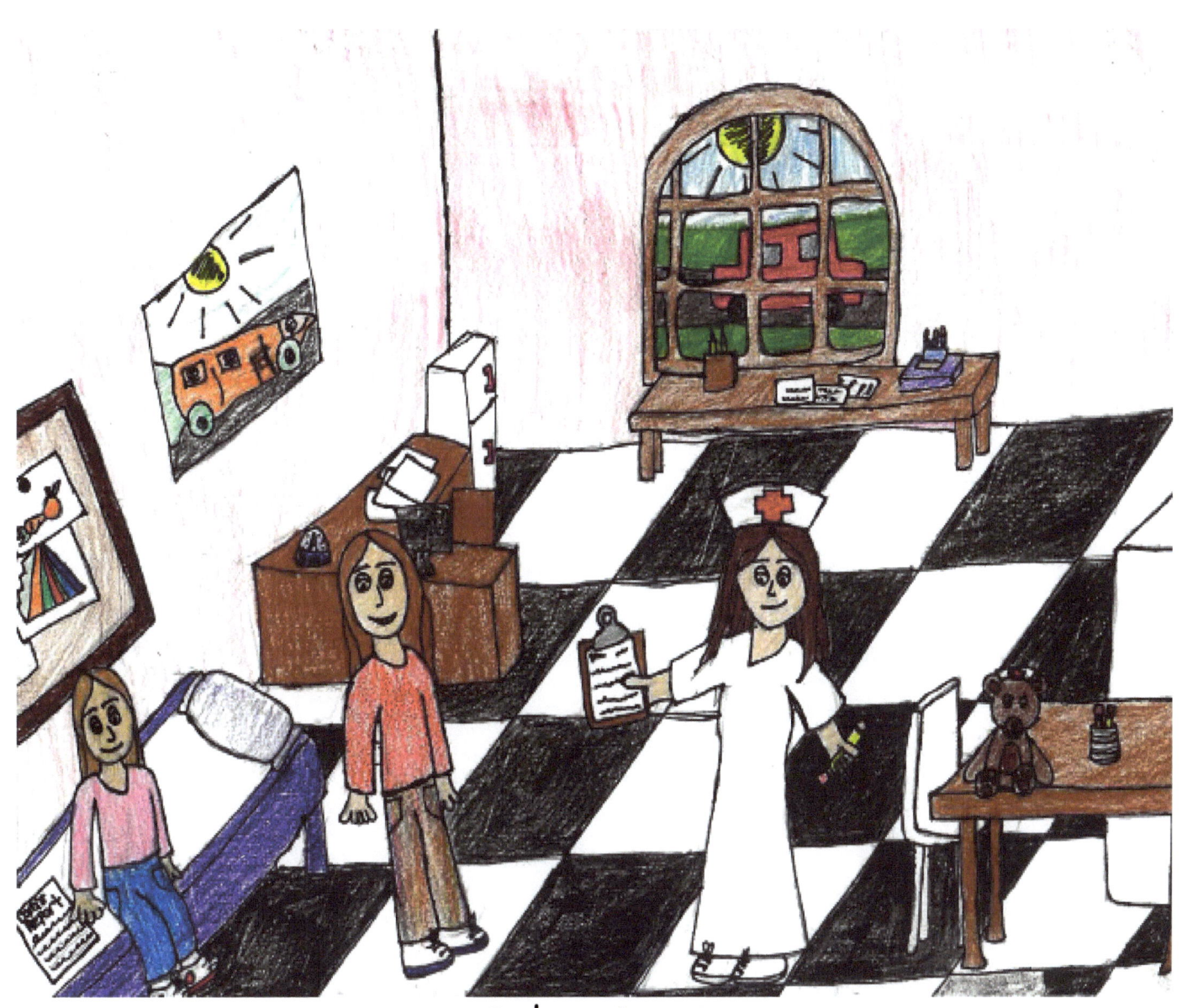

Sydney, Age 12
Allergic to fruit, sugar and dairy

After this story, Nurse Carewell told Dara and her mom more about epinephrine and reviewed with them how to use it if Dara ever had another allergic reaction. While Dara's mom practiced giving an injection (to an orange!), Dara and I watched and saw how easy it was.

Dara knew that even though epinephrine had to be given as a shot, she would need it to feel better. It wasn't scary at all!

As they left Nurse Carewell's office to go home, Dara smiled at her mom and sang "Food we never share, listen to Nurse Teddy Bear!"

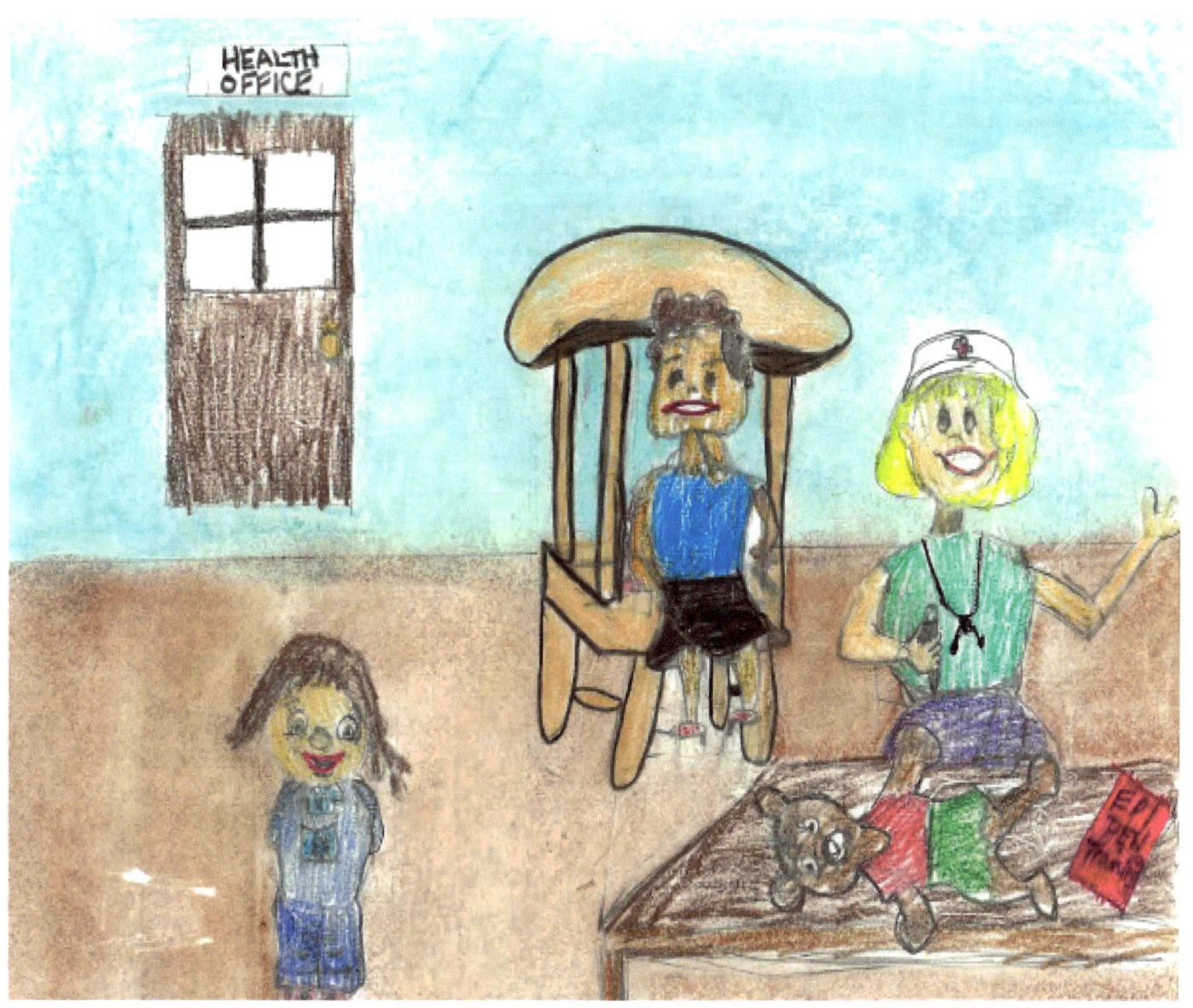

Trevor, Age 9
Allergic to walnuts, carrots and apples

As soon as we got back to Dara's house, her mom put out a snack of grapes and pretzels for us.

Dara asked her mom how she knew what foods she could eat. Her mom explained that she always checked the ingredients (all the parts in the food such as flour) to make sure her food did not contain peanuts or tree nuts.

Dara's mom reminded Dara never to eat a food unless she checked with her, Nurse Carewell or her teacher. She reassured Dara that the school lunches would be safe for her to eat.

She also said she would speak to Nurse Carewell often and that Nurse Carewell knew to check with Dara's mom if she had any questions or concerns. This made Dara and I feel much safer!!

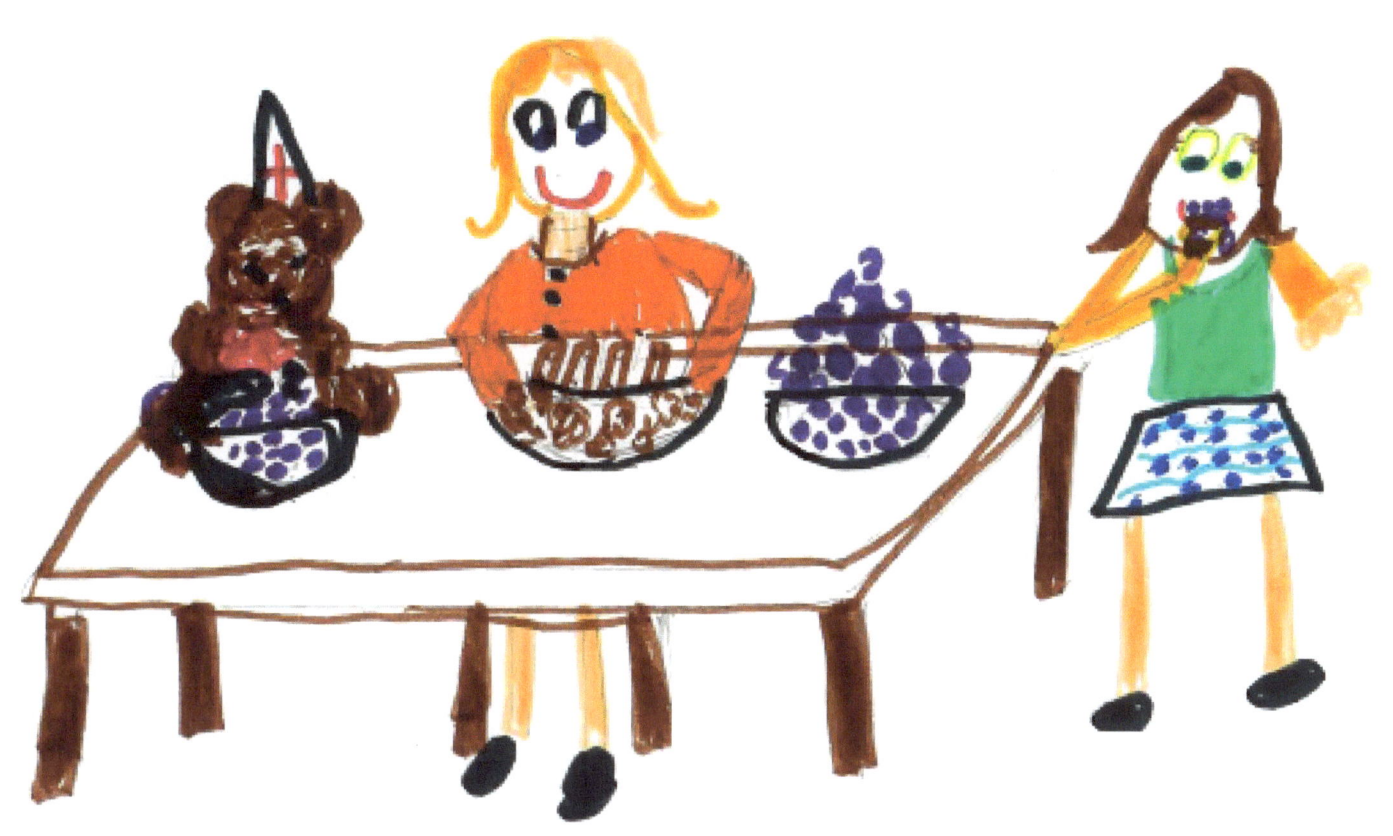

Meredith, Age 9
Allergic to tree nuts

My week spent with Dara went by very quickly. We did many fun things, and Dara taught me a lot about how she takes good care of herself in a healthy way.

Now I know all about healthy snacks, reading ingredient labels, and of course food allergies. I learned so much and can't wait to go home with another student and learn some more.

On Monday morning, Dara brought me back to class. We sang together "Food we never share, listen to Nurse Teddy Bear" and then she gave me a big hug and a kiss.

I'm going to miss Dara!

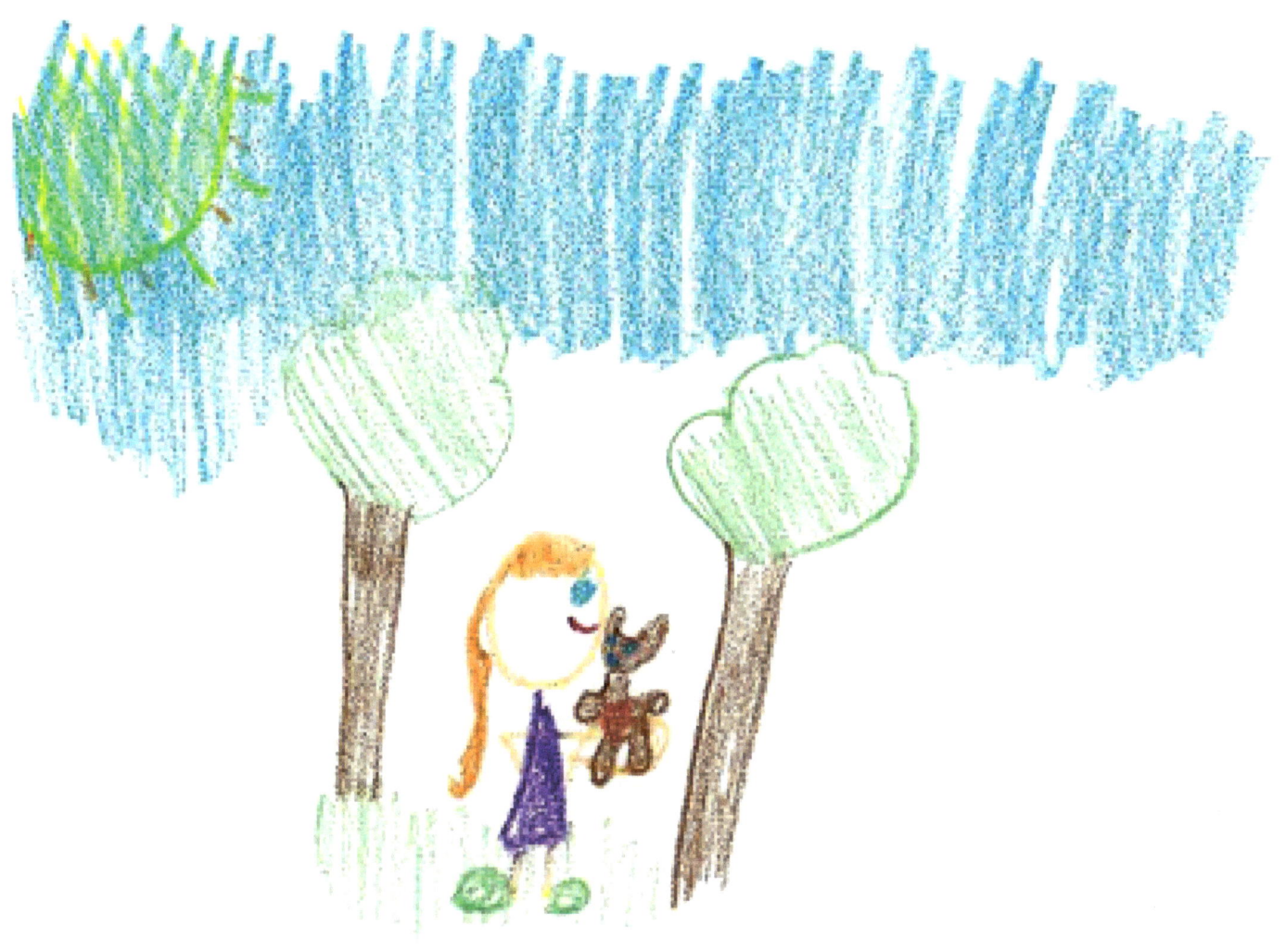

Ali, Age 7
Allergic to peanuts, tree nuts and shellfish

ACKNOWLEDGMENTS

I couldn't have put this book together without the help of many wonderful people including Cheryl Schwartz for her expert guidance and editing skill; Melinda Moses for her encouragement to write this book and her assistance in producing it; Dr. Zigelman, our school physician, for his professional guidance; all the parents who read this book and provided invaluable input and advice; and a huge thank you to my wonderful husband Dennis for his never-ending support.

And to all of the children who contributed their wonderful illustrations to these pages, Thank You! You have made this book extra special!

Some Interesting Facts About Food Allergies

- 1 in 25 children, including 6 - 8% of elementary students, have a food allergy. Here in New Jersey approximately 327,000 people have food allergies, including nearly 100,000 children.

- Eight foods account for 90% of allergic reactions. These include milk, eggs, peanuts, wheat, soy, tree nuts, fish, and shellfish.

- Symptoms of a reaction can include: a tingling sensation in the mouth; swelling of the lips, tongue, and throat; breathing difficulties; hives; vomiting; abdominal cramps; diarrhea; drop in blood pressure; loss of consciousness; and death. Symptoms can appear within seconds to hours after consuming the food to which one is allergic.

- Strict avoidance of allergy-causing foods is the only way to prevent a reaction. Reading the ingredient labels of all foods to be consumed and knowing the alternative names for allergens (such as "whey" and "casein" for milk) as well as preventing cross-contamination are the keys to minimizing allergic reactions.

- Food allergies are different from food intolerances. An intolerance is a metabolic disorder and does not involve the immune system. A food allergy occurs when the immune system reacts to a food protein causing symptoms that can affect the respiratory system, gastrointestinal tract, skin, and/or cardiovascular system.

Classroom Interventions and Celebrations Guidelines

Recommended that all classrooms designated as "Peanut/Tree nut Free" observe the following:

- All parents of students in Peanut/Tree Nut Free classrooms will be notified of the fact that there is at least 1 student in that particular class with a peanut/tree nut allergy.

- For daily snacks, do not send in any product containing peanuts, tree nuts (almonds, pecans, walnuts, cashews, pistachios, etc.) or their oils. Be sure to check all ingredient labels. Products labeled as "may contain nuts" or "produced in a facility that processes nuts" are not acceptable.

- Offer a Peanut/Tree Nut Free table to interested students with Peanut/Tree Nut allergies. If a student without such an allergy is invited to sit at this table, he or she must have a Peanut/Tree Nut Free lunch.

- For classroom celebrations, such as birthdays and holiday parties, all food must be in its original container with the nutrition label intact. All food must be brought to the nurse's office for approval prior to entering the classroom.

- All parents of students with food allergies are encouraged to send in a supply of safe snacks for their children. These will be served when the classroom celebration treat is unsafe or when prohibited by the parents.

- Students with food allergies may not eat any homemade food items from other homes.

- Students with food allergies may eat food that has been approved by the nurse only with prior parental permission. If there are any safety concerns whatsoever, the food will not be served and the student will have one of the safe snacks that have been provided by his or her parent(s).

- Students can have a variety of food allergies including dairy, egg, wheat, soy, sesame, fruit, vegetables, food coloring, etc. Although only peanuts and tree nuts are prohibited, please remember that the nurse considers numerous factors when assessing the safety of food before it enters a classroom and that is the reason for final approval.

- Although foods may be approved by the nurse, please remember that the final decision to serve the food to the food allergic student rests with his or her own parent(s).

- If parents or teachers choose to distribute goody bags, they must contain non-edible items.

- Students are advised to wash their hands before and after consuming food.

- Students are not allowed to share or swap food.

- There are several days throughout the school year when students will eat their lunches in the classrooms (Election Day, Book Fair, etc.). Prior notice will be sent home with the students in Peanut/Tree Nut Free classrooms and also will be posted on the school website. On these days, lunches brought to school must be free of peanuts, tree nuts, and their oils.

- For some suggestions regarding safe foods, please consult www.SnackSafely.com. Please note that these foods still require approval by the nurse since labeling changes are common.

- All classroom activities and holiday projects must use non-edible items.

General Nutritional Snack Guidelines

- Snacks should contain no more than 8 grams of total fat per serving, and no more than 2 grams of saturated fat per serving. Sugar cannot be the first ingredient.

- All beverages shall not exceed 12 oz., except water or milk containing 2% or less fat.

- Suggested snacks include: fruit, vegetables, pretzels, cheese & crackers, and yogurt.

Cafeteria Interventions

- All foods served in the school cafeteria are free of peanuts and tree nuts.

- An allergen-free table will be an available option for all allergic students.

- Students are not allowed to share or swap food.

- Students are advised to wash their hands before and after consuming food.

- If there is a need for a peanut/tree nut free table and a student without food allergies is invited to sit there, he or she must have a peanut/tree nut free lunch on that day.

- Additional interventions may be implemented to meet individual student needs.

Field Trip Guidelines

- A school nurse or trained delegate will be available during all school-sponsored field trips.

- Parents of the food allergic students are encouraged, but not required, to accompany their children on field trips.

- In an effort to promote the health and safety of all students, eating on the bus is strongly discouraged.

- The appropriateness of all field trips will be evaluated in consideration of the needs of all students. For example, a trip to a dairy farm would not be scheduled for a class with a milk-allergic student.

REFERENCES

- American Academy of Pediatrics, *www.aap.org*

- Food Allergy Research and Education, *www.foodallergy.org*

- National Association of School Nurses, *www.nasn.org*

- New Jersey State Department of Education, *www.state.nj.us*

- SnackSafely.com, *www.SnackSafely.com*

- Allergy and Asthma Network, *www.aanma.org*

- New York State Department of Health, *www.health.state.ny.us*

- Hillsdale Public School District, *www.hillsdaleschools.com*

- Kids with Food Allergies, www.kidswithfoodallergies.org

RESOURCES

- American Academy of Pediatrics, *www.aap.org*

- Food Allergy Research and Education, *www.foodallergy.org*

- National Association of School Nurses, *www.nasn.org*

- New Jersey State Department of Education, *www.state.nj.us*

- SnackSafely.com, *www.SnackSafely.com*

- Allergy and Asthma Network, *www.aanma.org*

- Kids with Food Allergies, www.kidswithfoodallergies.org

About the Author

Ann Lempert Deutsch,
RN, MSN, CPNP

Ann Deutsch has over 35 years of nursing experience, 17 of those years working as an elementary school nurse. She enjoys educating children, parents and the school community about food allergies, and hopes this book will be used to help all teachers, children and families be better informed and sensitive about food allergies. Ann is married with two children of her own.

A very special thanks to all of the talented children from Ann's school who contributed their wonderful illustrations to this book.

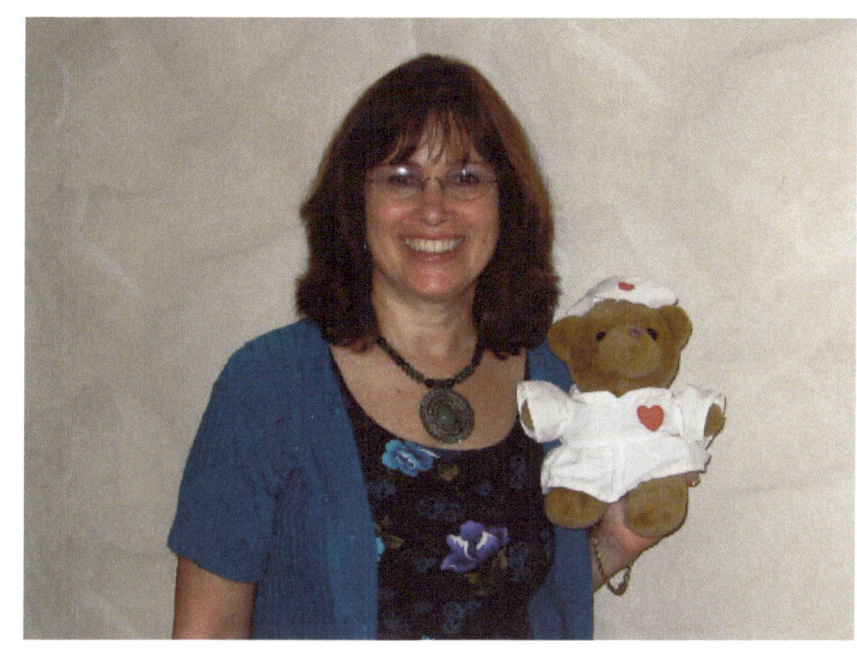